The Sensuous Heart

guidelines for sex after heart attack or heart surgery

by Suzanne Cambre, RN, BSHA
Cardiology Nurse

Do not use this book to replace the advice and treatment you get from your doctor. This book is only to support what you already know about having sex after a heart attack or heart surgery.

Contents

If you enjoyed sex before your heart attack or heart surgery, you can enjoy it afterwards.

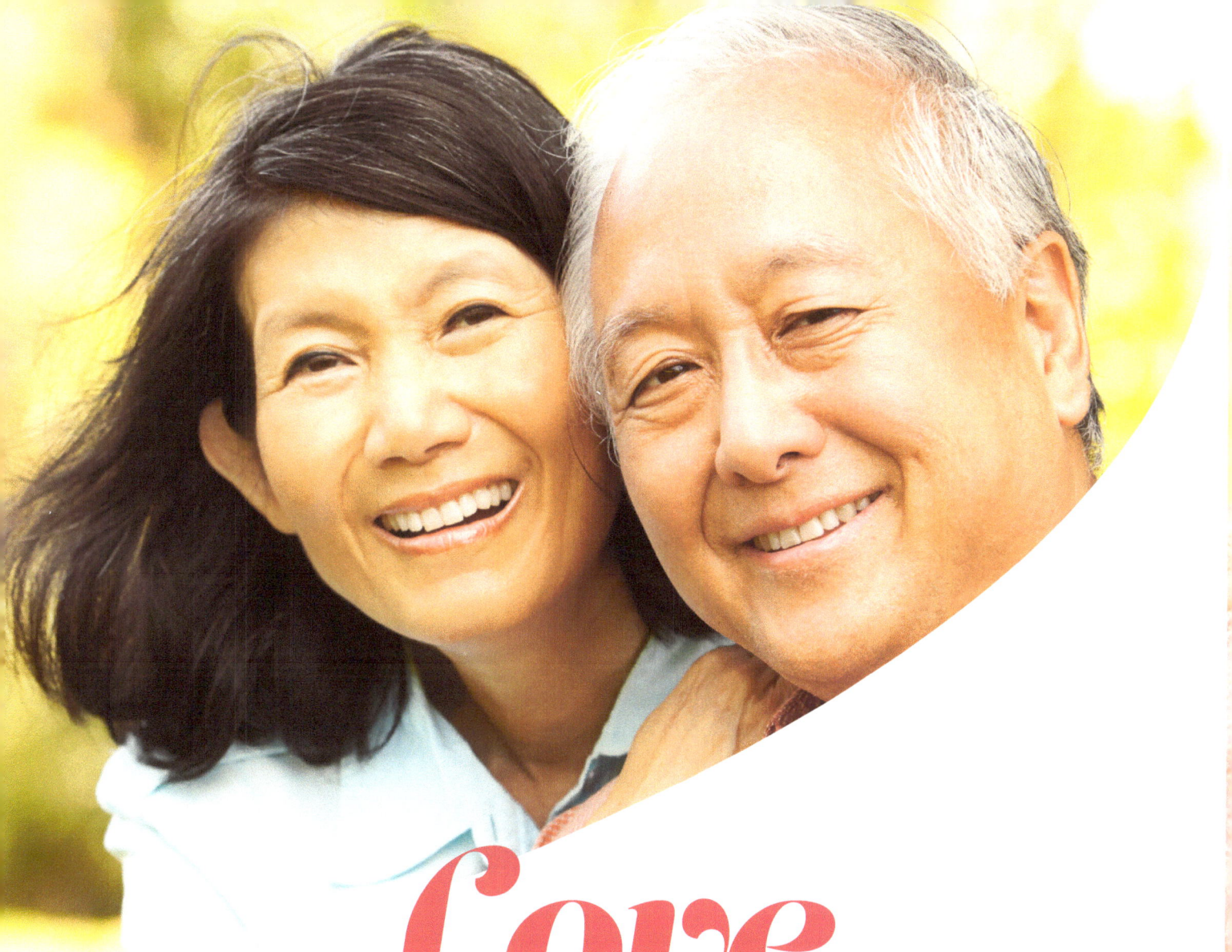

Love

For ages, the heart has been the symbol of love, tenderness and caring. Yet when the heart is damaged, little is said about getting back to the act of loving – sexual intercourse. Since little is said, one may think the worst.

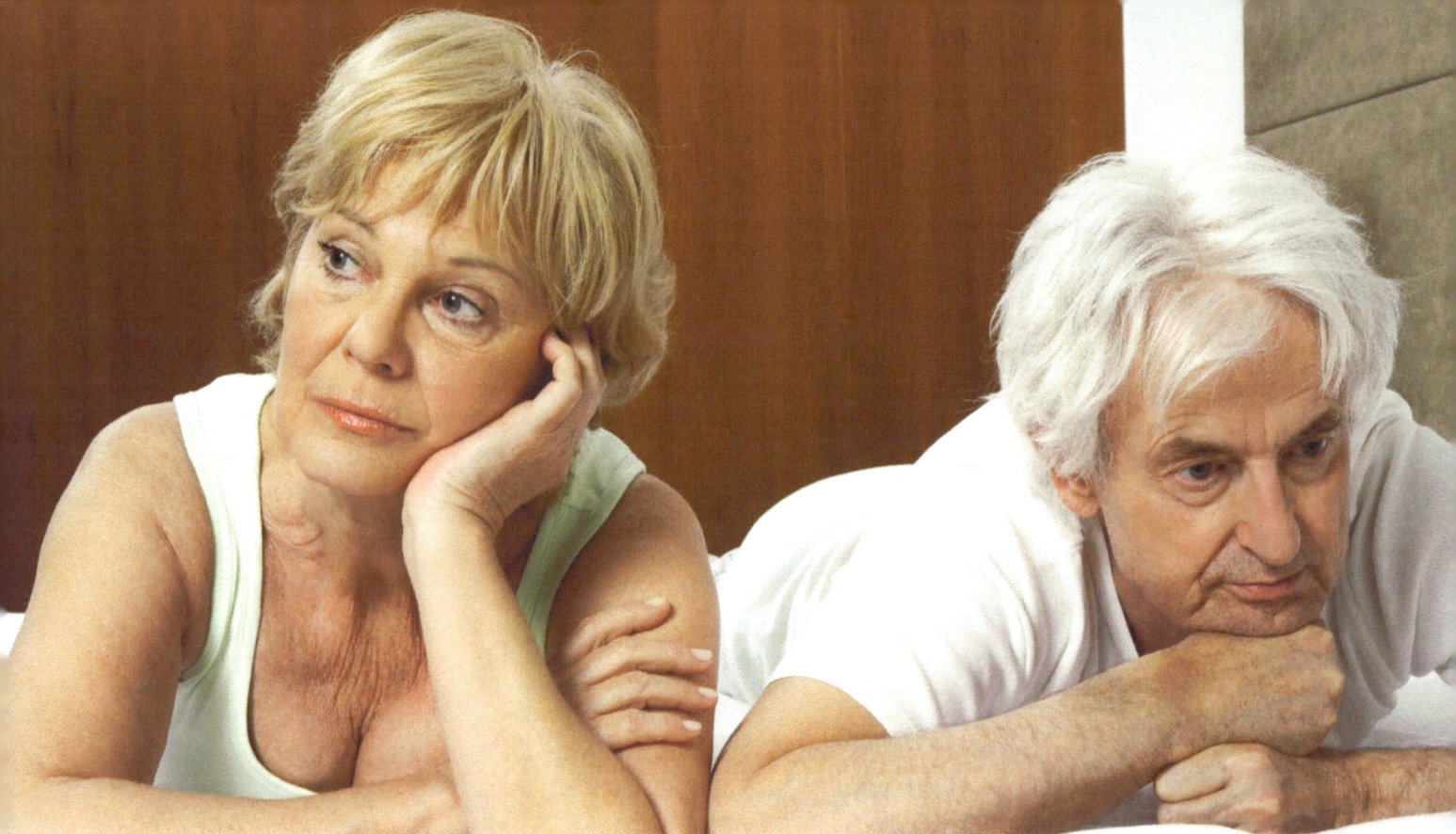

Sex after a heart attack

After having a heart attack, many fear that their sex life is over. They think that sex will put too much stress on a damaged heart. Movies and books often feed this fear. They are full of scenes where the person who has a heart problem dies in the arms of a loved one. There is even a legend that Attila the Hun died during sex, not during battle. Patients and doctors add to these fears when they are not open and frank about sex.

Most people who have an uncomplicated heart attack return to their usual activities. This includes a return to sex usually within several weeks after the heart attack*. So you see, sex is not as risky for your heart as you might think. As a matter of fact, the number of heart attacks brought on by physical effort is fairly low.

* People with complicated heart attacks (serious rhythm problems, blood pressure problems or heart muscle weakness) may take a longer time to heal.

Sex after heart surgery

If you had heart surgery (but not a heart attack), you can have sex soon afterwards. How soon will depend on the healing of the breastbone and chest incision. You may want to postpone sex until your chest feels less sore, but this is up to you. It most often takes 4 to 6 weeks after surgery to get your strength back and about the same time for the breastbone to mend.

Recovery will not be the same for each person. How fast a person recovers depends on the extent of the surgery and the type of medicines taken.

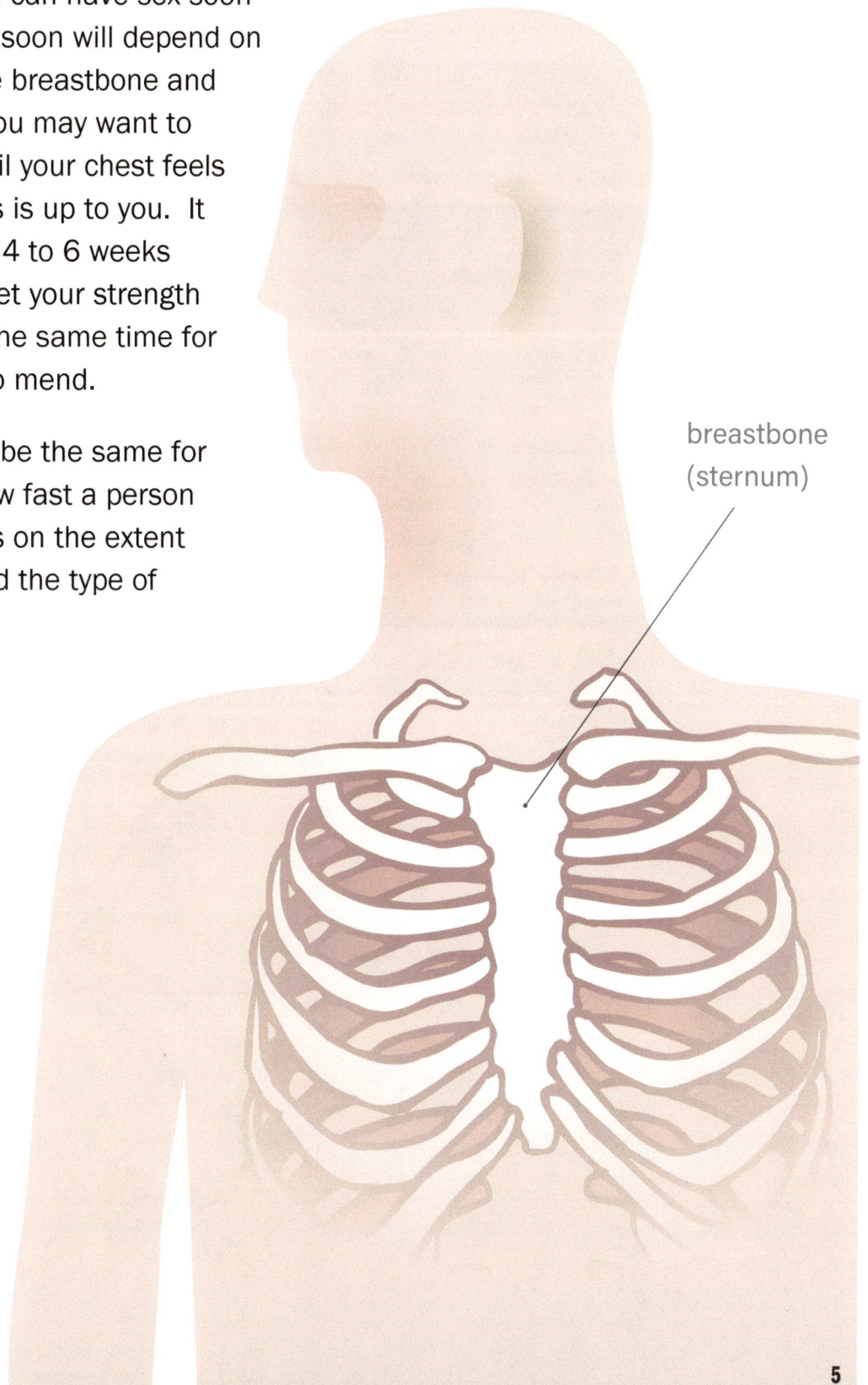

breastbone
(sternum)

Sex after heart cath or angioplasty

In the absence of a heart attack, there is no restriction about sex after a cardiac cath or balloon procedure. You will only need to wait until the puncture site has closed and there is no significant swelling or drainage. 24 hours is the usual time.

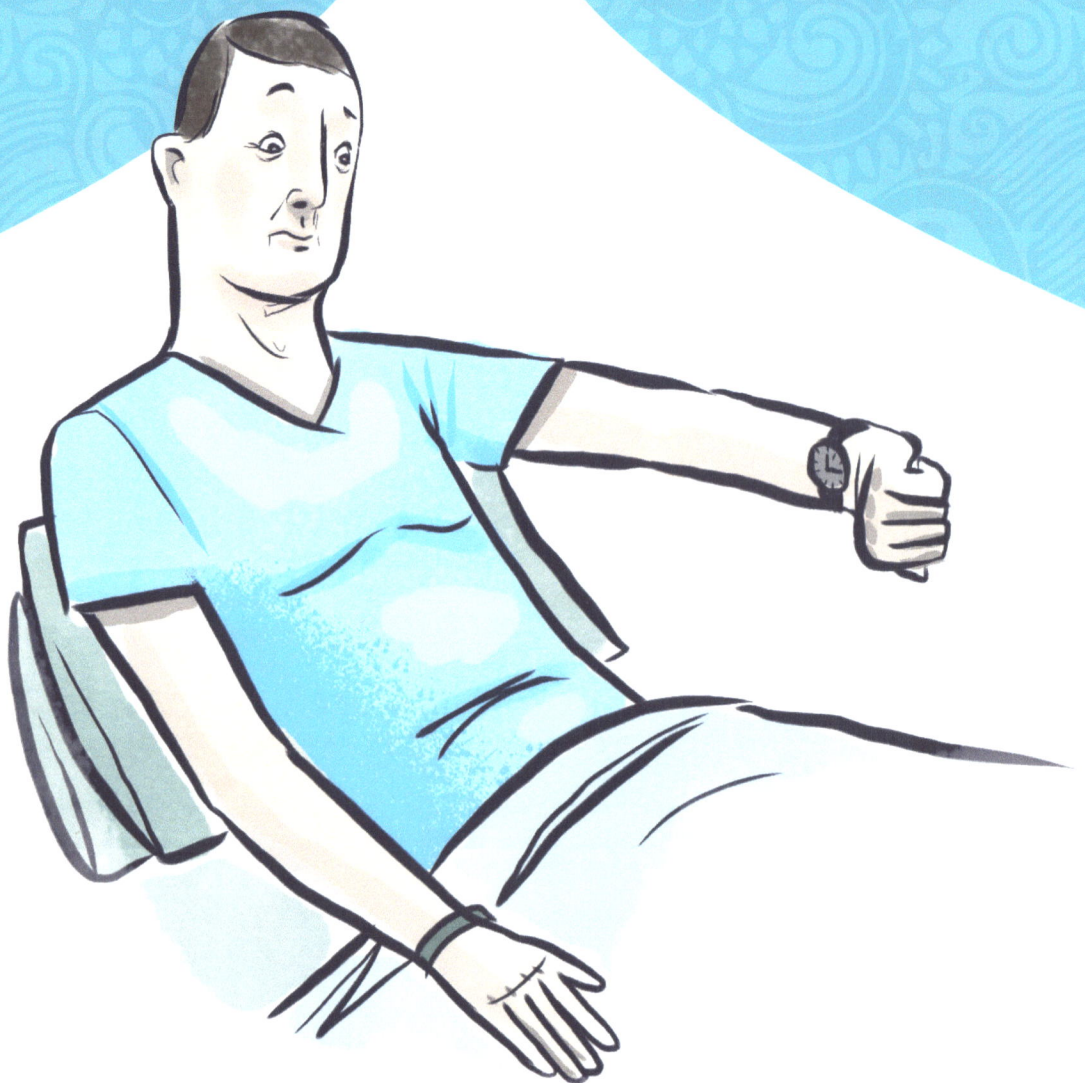

Getting in touch again

Hugs and kisses are warm ways to get back in touch with your partner. This is true after any separation such as that caused by an illness.

After a heart attack or surgery, simple touching helps you begin slowly and work up in stages. It helps you feel wanted and close to your partner.

Don't feel that every hug must lead to sex. Don't set goals for each other such as, "We have to do it every day," or "If I don't have orgasm, sex isn't good." This can add stress to sex and make you too uptight to enjoy it.

Do what makes you feel relaxed and good. Remember, love can be expressed in many ways besides sex.

Feeling depressed

It is common for one or both partners to feel tired or depressed after one has a heart attack or heart surgery. This can cause less desire for sex. You may both be thinking, "Can we even have sex?" or "Will sex be any good?" If you feel blue and are thinking these things, talk about them. Both partners have to rebuild their sex life.

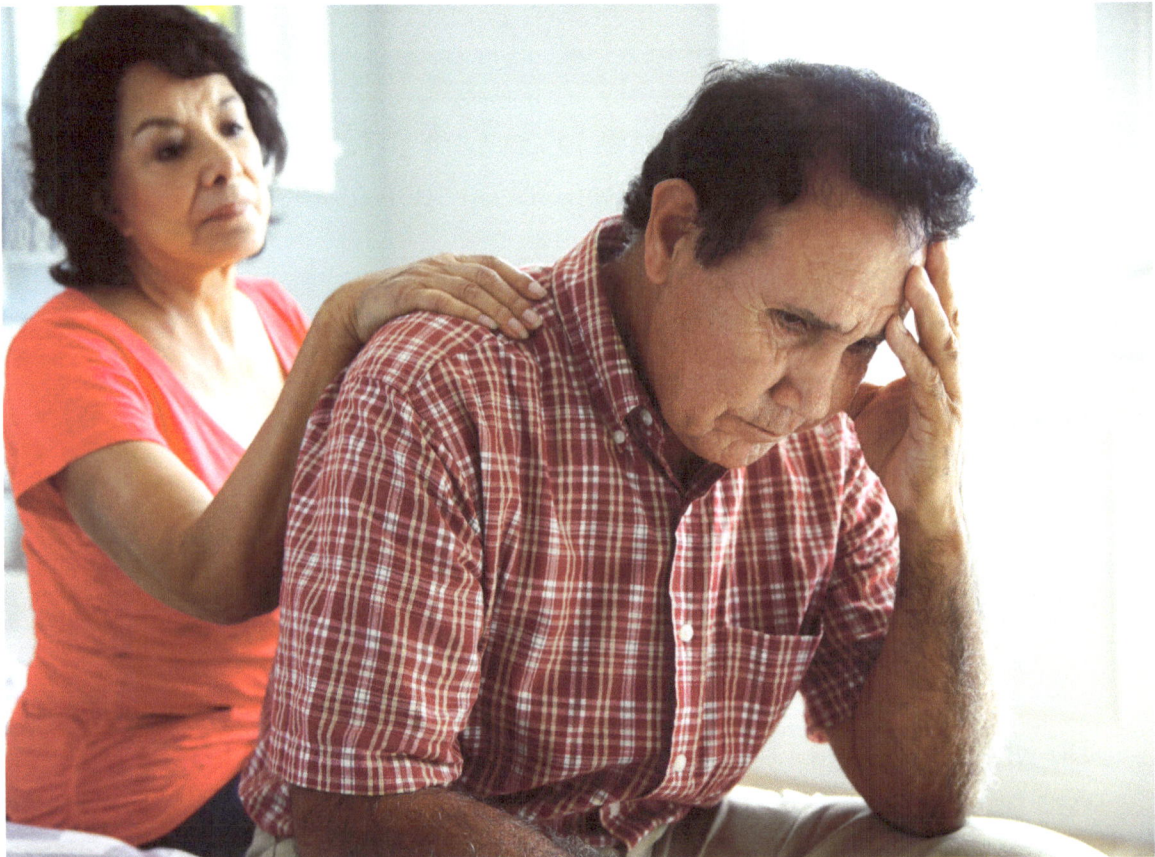

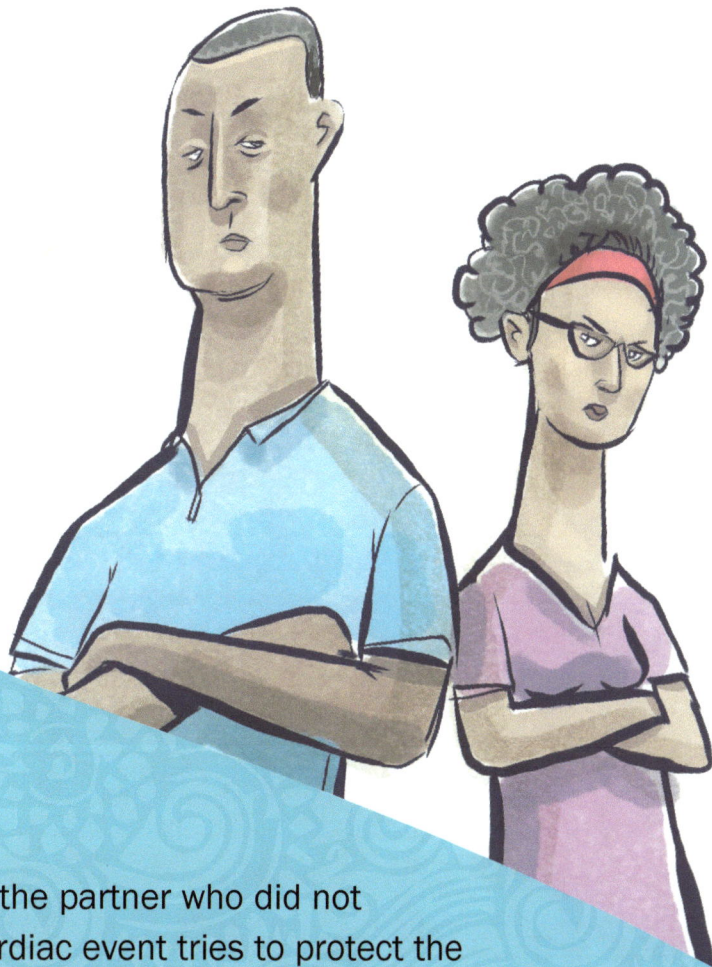

Sometimes the partner who did not have the cardiac event tries to protect the one who did. This is normal when a loved one is ill. Yet, you may feel like a "cripple," "put down," angry or guilty. If you do not talk about these feelings, they can hurt a relationship and interfere with sex. Anger in itself can be a trigger for an increased risk of cardiac events.

In today's world, it's more common for people to discuss sex with friends, family and their doctors. There is not as much shyness about this as in years past. So don't be embarrassed to ask your doctor or nurse about sex. Express your feelings. Sharing can make the road to recovery a lot less bumpy.

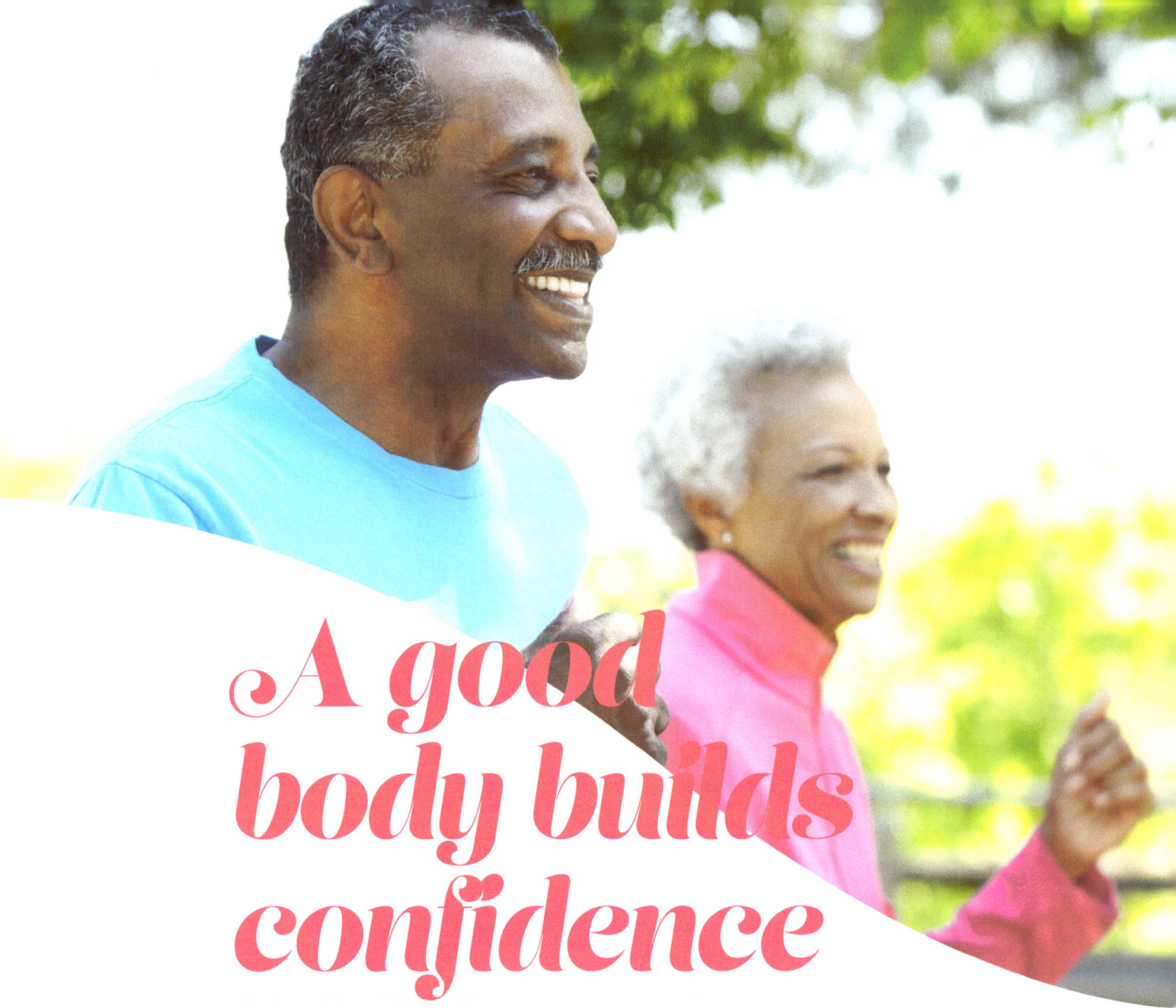

A good body builds confidence

After a heart attack or surgery, your body is out of shape. To help you get back your strength many doctors prescribe gradual exercises. These could be:

- **walking**

- **swimming**

- **golf with a cart**

- **home treadmill or stationary bike**

Exercise is one of the best cures for "the blues". It also helps you feel less dependent and more at ease about what your body can do.

Exercise can help the heart do the same amount of work with less effort. The first step is to **check with your doctor before starting any form of exercise.** You may be given a stress test to find out how much you can do. Some people find supervised exercise in a cardiac rehab program helpful. Ask your doctor about such a program in your area. Insurance covers most rehab programs.

Keep in mind that the type and amount of exercise you do will depend on your age and fitness level.

Note

Start slow. Build up as you go.

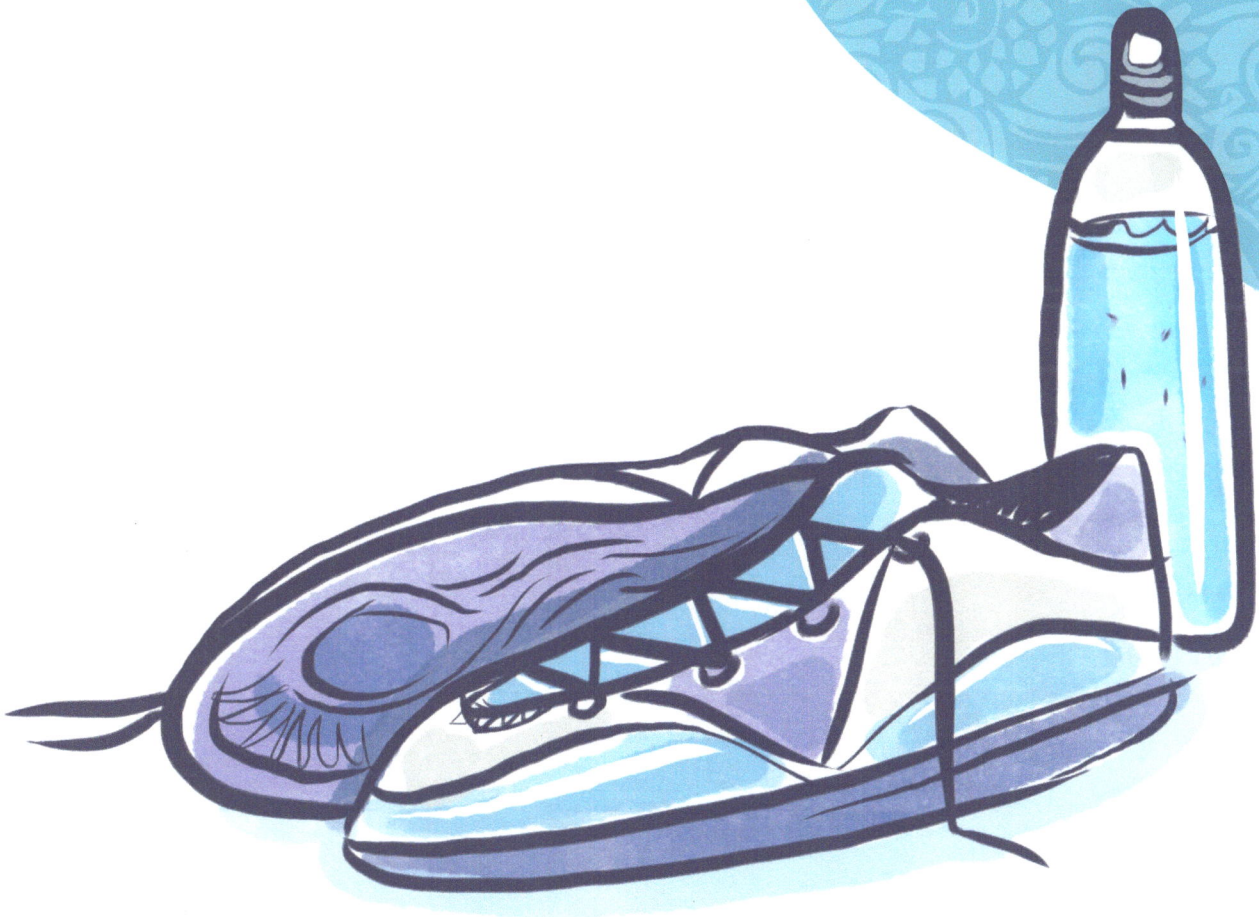

Read on if you're ready for more...

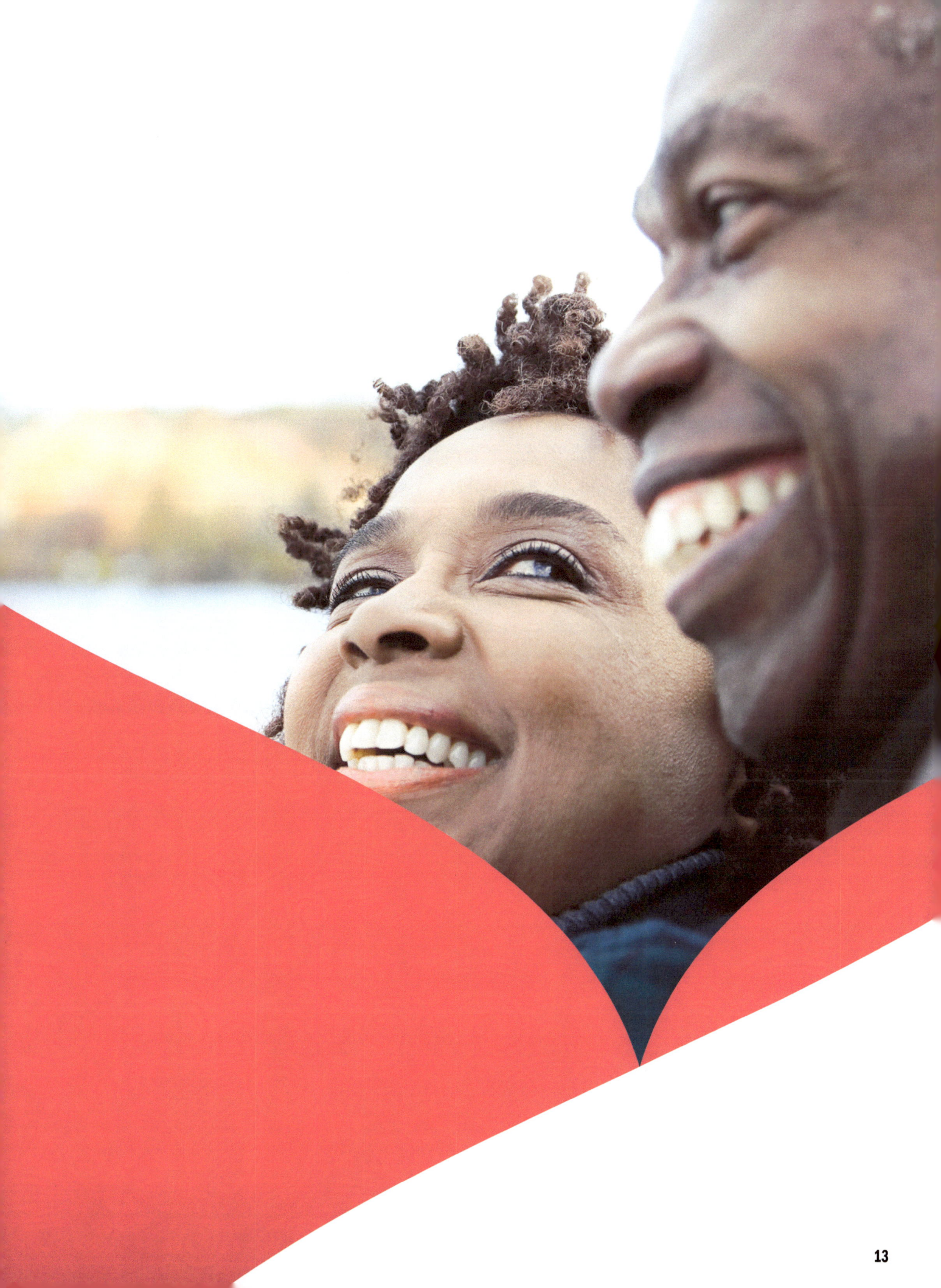

Your body during sex

Many activities can raise your heart rate. Climbing stairs and walking are two of the most common. During these, your heart beats from 107 to 130 times a minute. During sex, your heart beats about 117 times a minute.

If you don't get short of breath, have chest pain or get tired when climbing two flights of stairs or doing something like it, your heart can meet the demands needed for sex.

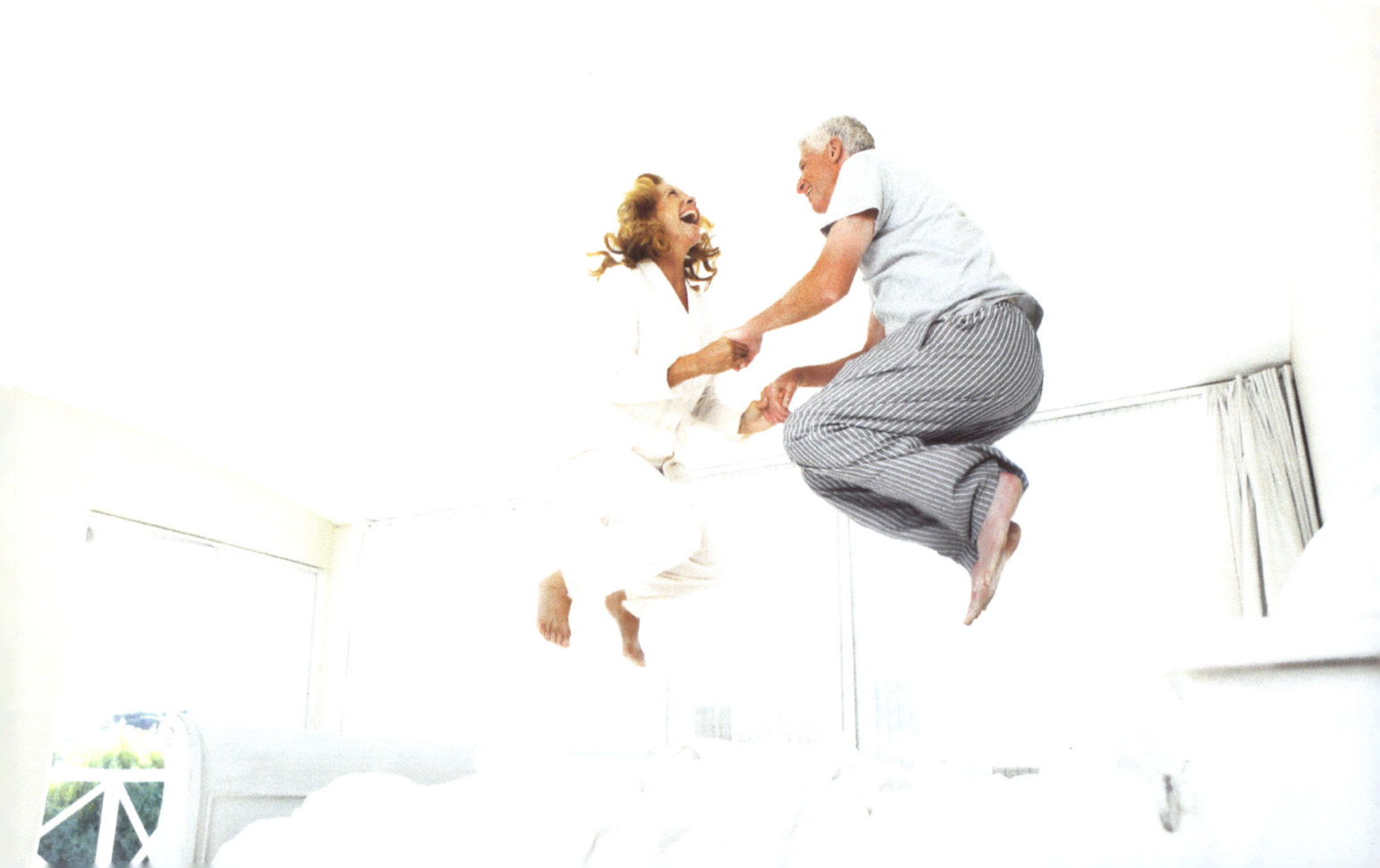

Four phases of sexual activity

Your body changes
in these ways during sex:

arousal 1. skin becomes flushed;
breathing and pulse rate increase;
blood pressure is up slightly

plateau 2. an increase in the above signs

orgasm 3. the heart works hardest here;
pulse rate may reach 150 beats
or more per minute; blood pressure
may exceed 160/90; this phase lasts
15-20 seconds

resolution 4. body returns to a resting pulse rate
and blood pressure within a matter of
seconds; angina or palpitations (a fast
or irregular heartbeat) happen most
often in this phase (if at all)

Call your doctor if palpitations last longer than 15
minutes after sex. Your doctor should also be aware of
lengthy chest discomfort, trouble breathing or unusual
extreme tiredness after having sex.

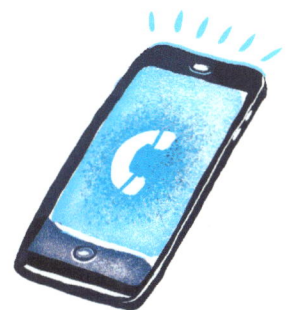

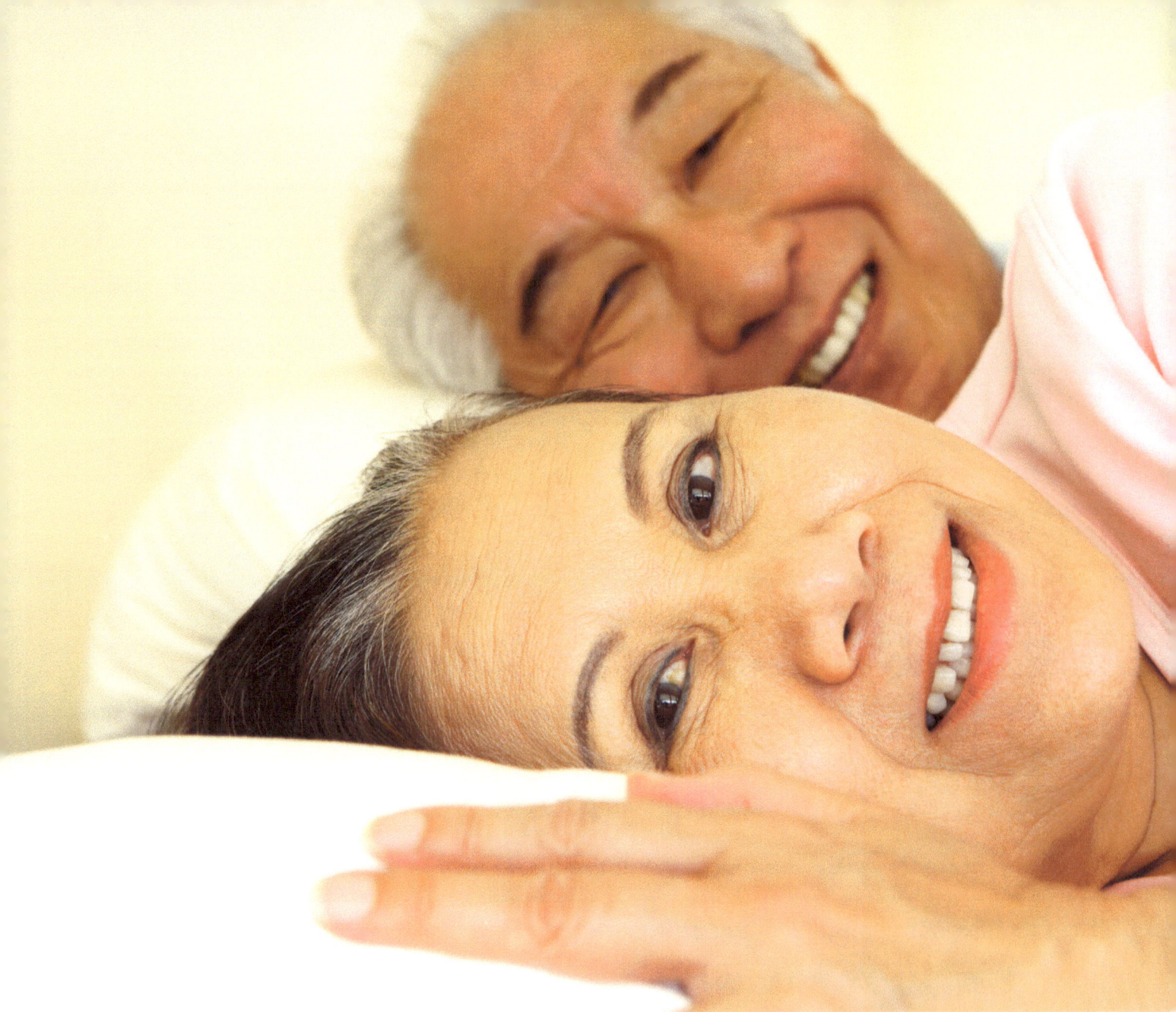

For most people, the time used to have sex is fairly short. The average middle-aged person having sex with the same partner twice a week has a total time from arousal to resolution of 10 to 16 minutes. During this time, **the greatest stress on the heart lasts only 4 to 6 minutes.**

How often you have sex

How often you have sex depends mostly on what your habits were before the cardiac event. If the sex you enjoyed before was without stress, use that as your guide. The idea that someone needs to have a lot of sex or sex with new partners to prove that he or she is "OK" is not true.

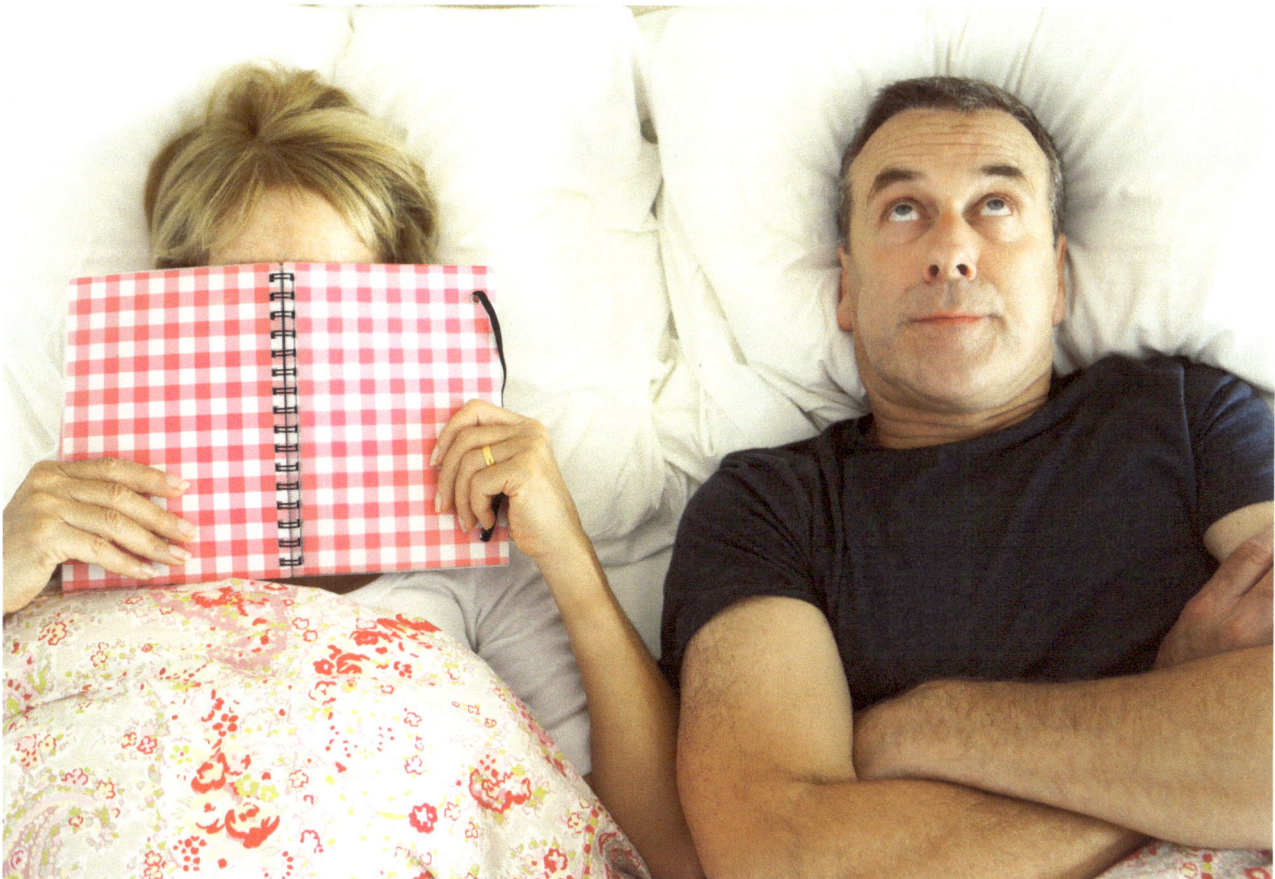

Get yourself ready

If you feel good about what your body can do and want to have sex, work up to it slowly. Sexual foreplay in a relaxed place helps you to get in the mood for sex. It also lets your heart rate and blood pressure increase more slowly.

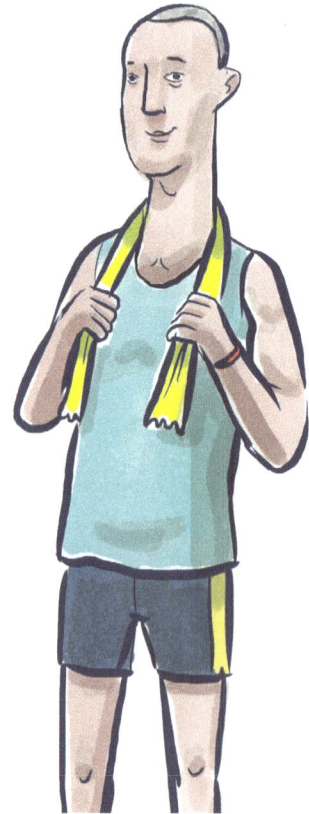

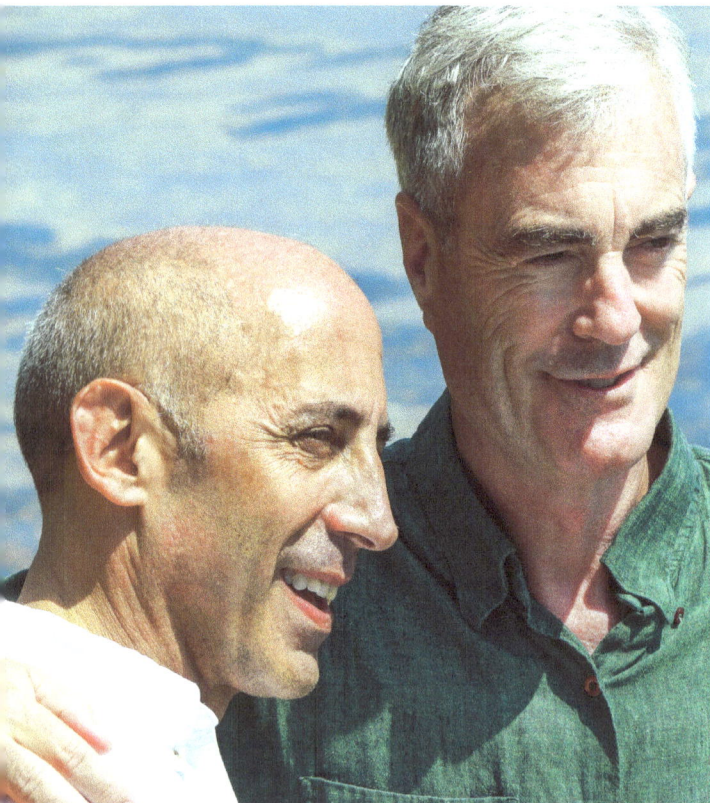

Other choices

The effects on the heart of masturbation and manual or oral stimulation are similar to intercourse.

Anal intercourse* or stimulation may lead to slower than normal heart rates and decreased blood flow to the heart muscle. Do not do this unless you clear it with your doctor.

* Persons at risk for acquiring the HIV/AIDS virus should practice "safe sex". Ask your doctor or go to the internet and research "safe sex education" for additional information.

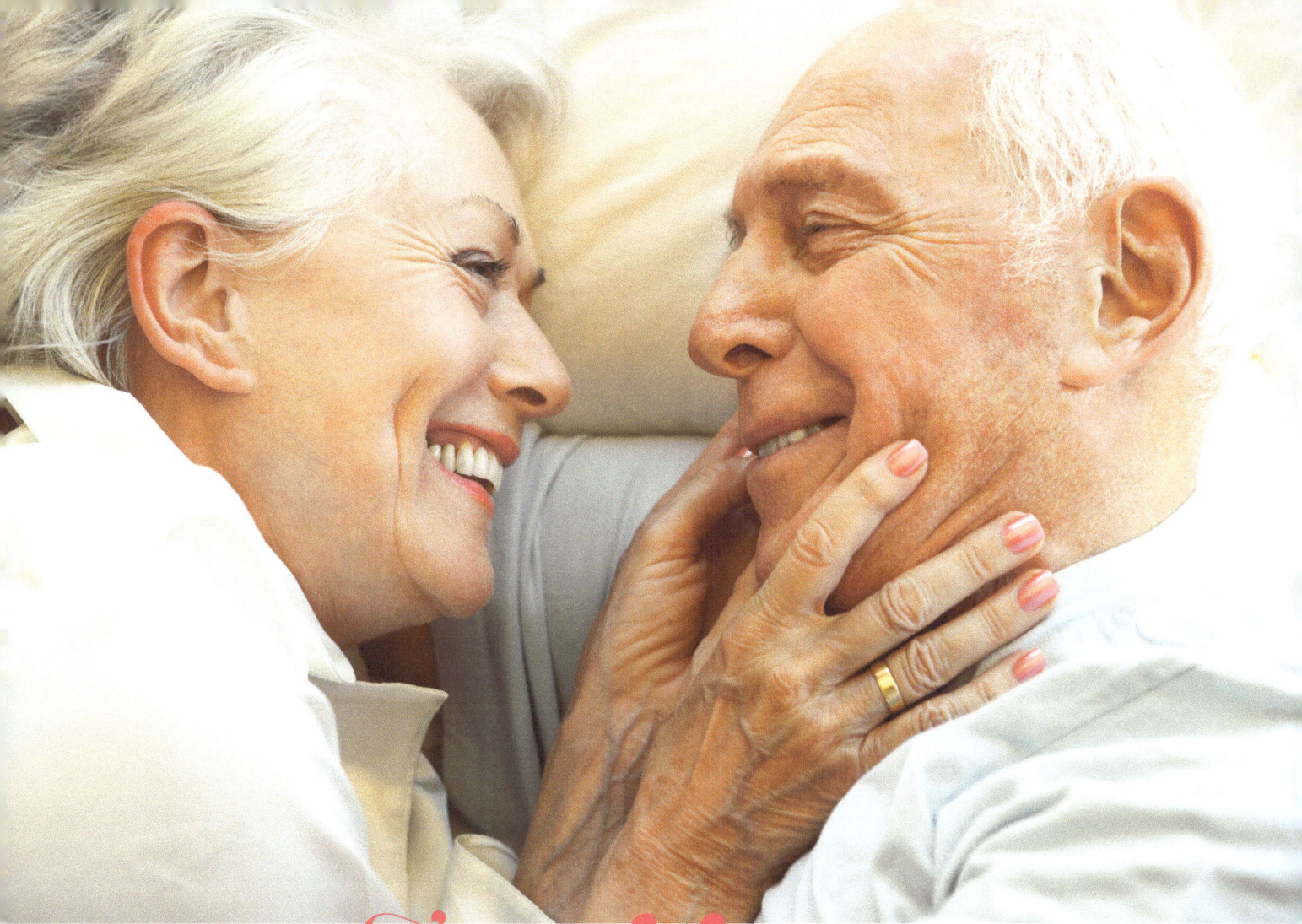

Positions

The person who had the cardiac event should **avoid sex positions that keep him or her on the arms for a long time. This is more true after heart surgery.** Using the arms for support pulls on the healing chest.

Some people find that sex is easier when both partners are **lying on their sides.** They can face each other or lie one behind the other. Others find it easier **sitting** face-to-face.

No major changes in sex positions should be tried if changes make either partner tired or anxious. Anxiety and fatigue can cause more work for your heart.

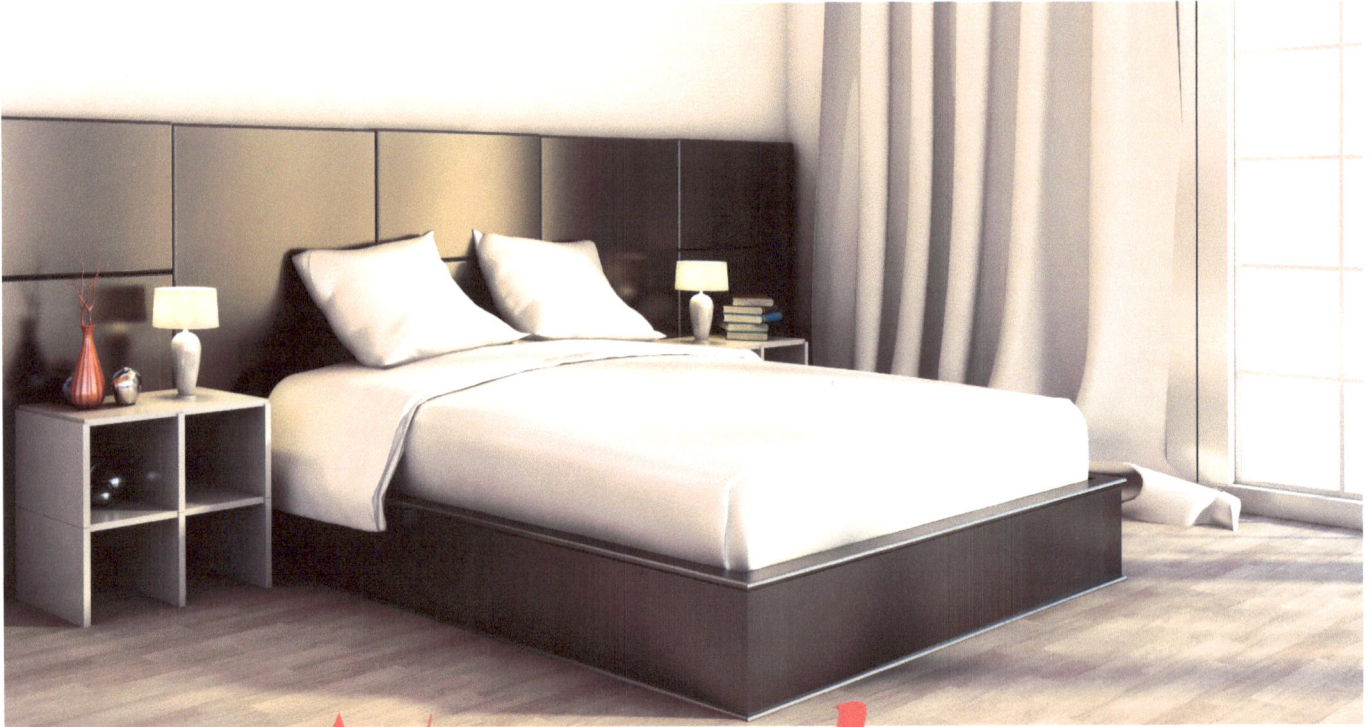

Atmosphere

When you are angry, stressed or tired, postpone sex. At these times your heart already beats faster. Sex would be an added strain.

Have sex in a pleasant place. Be comfortable. For example, if you are cold because its 50° inside or hot because you are smothered in blankets, you won't be relaxed.

Don't take very hot or cold baths, showers, saunas or whirlpool baths just before having sex. These cause a change in blood pressure as blood vessels open or close with extreme heat or cold.

Be rested before sex. Keep in mind that you shouldn't change your habits if this makes you anxious.

Eating and Drinking

Food and drink are other ways of sharing and saying, "I love you." But if you have had a heart attack, **don't have sex right after a heavy meal.**

Your heart will be sending extra blood to the stomach to help digest the food. Wait at least an hour for sex and other forms of exercise.

Excess alcohol can be dangerous to the heart and decrease sexual arousal. Men should limit alcohol to two drinks a day (women, one drink). Also, ask your doctor if alcohol might cause side effects with any medicine(s) that you are taking. **People with a drinking problem should avoid alcohol.**

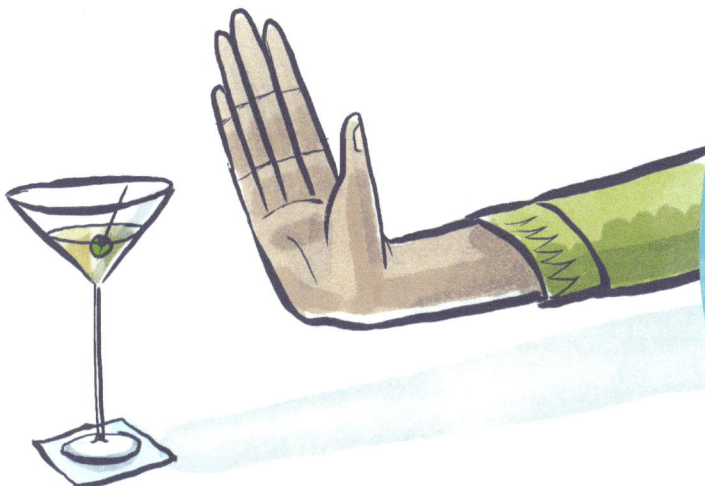

Note

One drink is:

one 12 oz beer
or
4 oz of wine
or
1½ oz of 80 proof liquor (or 1 oz of 100 proof)

Medicines

Some medicines used to treat coronary disease or high blood pressure may cause a decrease in sex drive or cause difficulty with erections. If you are having problems, talk with your doctor or nurse to see if these medicines can be changed or the dose reduced.

You may have angina during sex just as you may with other activities. If this occurs, take nitroglycerin and rest for a while before going on with sex. If the pain does not go away or comes back often, let your doctor know. Some people take a NTG before sex to help prevent angina **(Caution: this may cause a drop in blood pressure).**

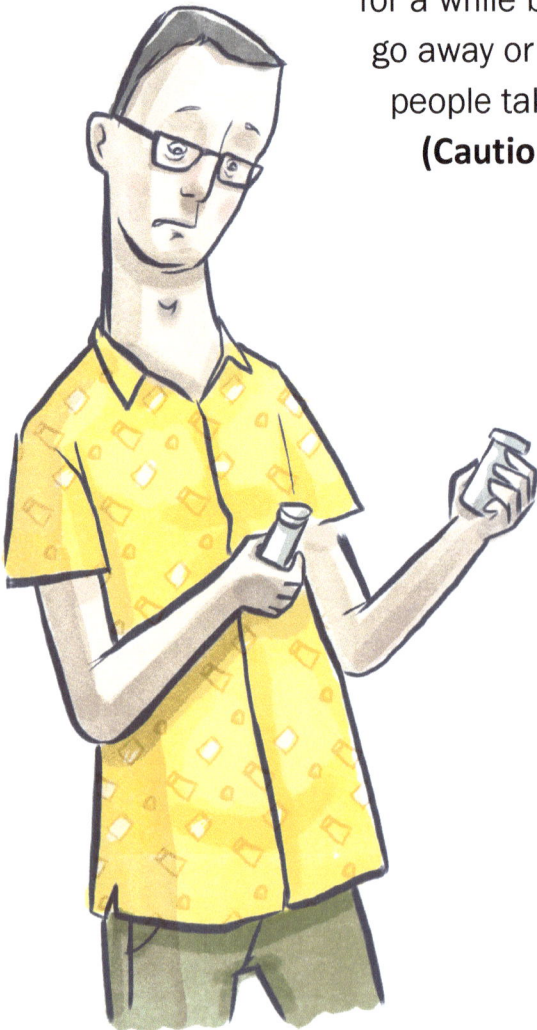

ED (erectile dysfunction) drugs like Viagra® Cialis® and Levitra® can cause dangerous drops in blood pressure if taken within 24 hours of any form of nitroglycerin. This includes nitroglycerin pills, patches, sprays and amyl nitrate "poppers". Other drugs like those used for high pressures in the lungs (Revatio® and Adcirca®) have the same 24 hour restrictions for nitro use. **If you have symptoms** for which you would normally use nitroglycerin **and you have used any of the above drugs** within a 24 hour period, **do not use the nitro.** Go to the nearest ER for treatment. You should always tell your doctor all the medications you are taking including over the counter medication and "herbal remedies" so that any problems can be avoided.

Women with heart disease may be asked not to use birth control pills. The woman who wishes to become pregnant should first talk to her doctor. Starting hormone replacement therapy (HRT) after a heart attack or cardiac event **might be harmful.** The continued use of HRT is a decision that must be made with a doctor familiar with your heart history.

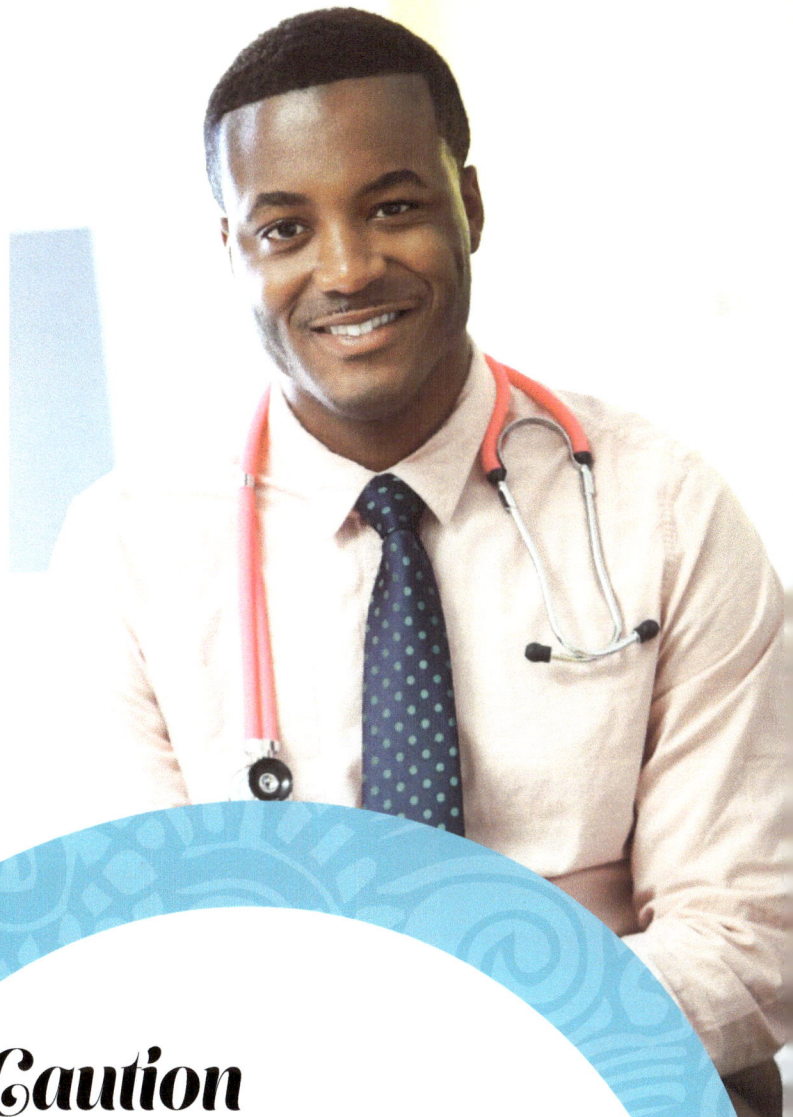

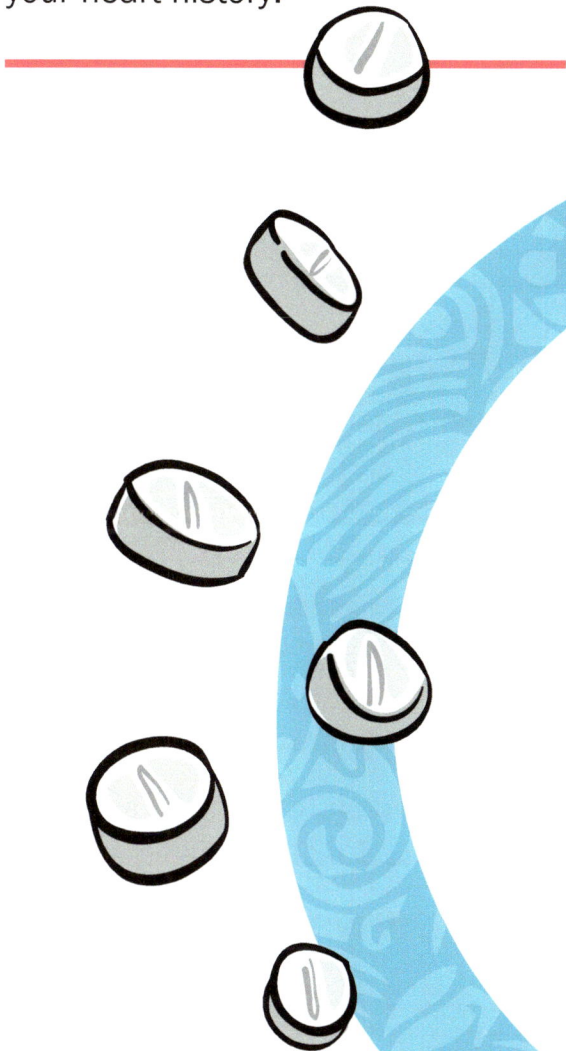

Caution

Stimulants (like amphetamines or amyl nitrate "poppers") may be dangerous. **Herbals containing ephedra (herbal ecstasy), Yohimbe and Siberian Ginseng** may have dangerous effects on the heart. **Marijuana** raises the heart rate and oxygen needs of the heart muscle. **Cocaine** can cause fatal heart attacks. These drugs are harmful and **should not be used.**

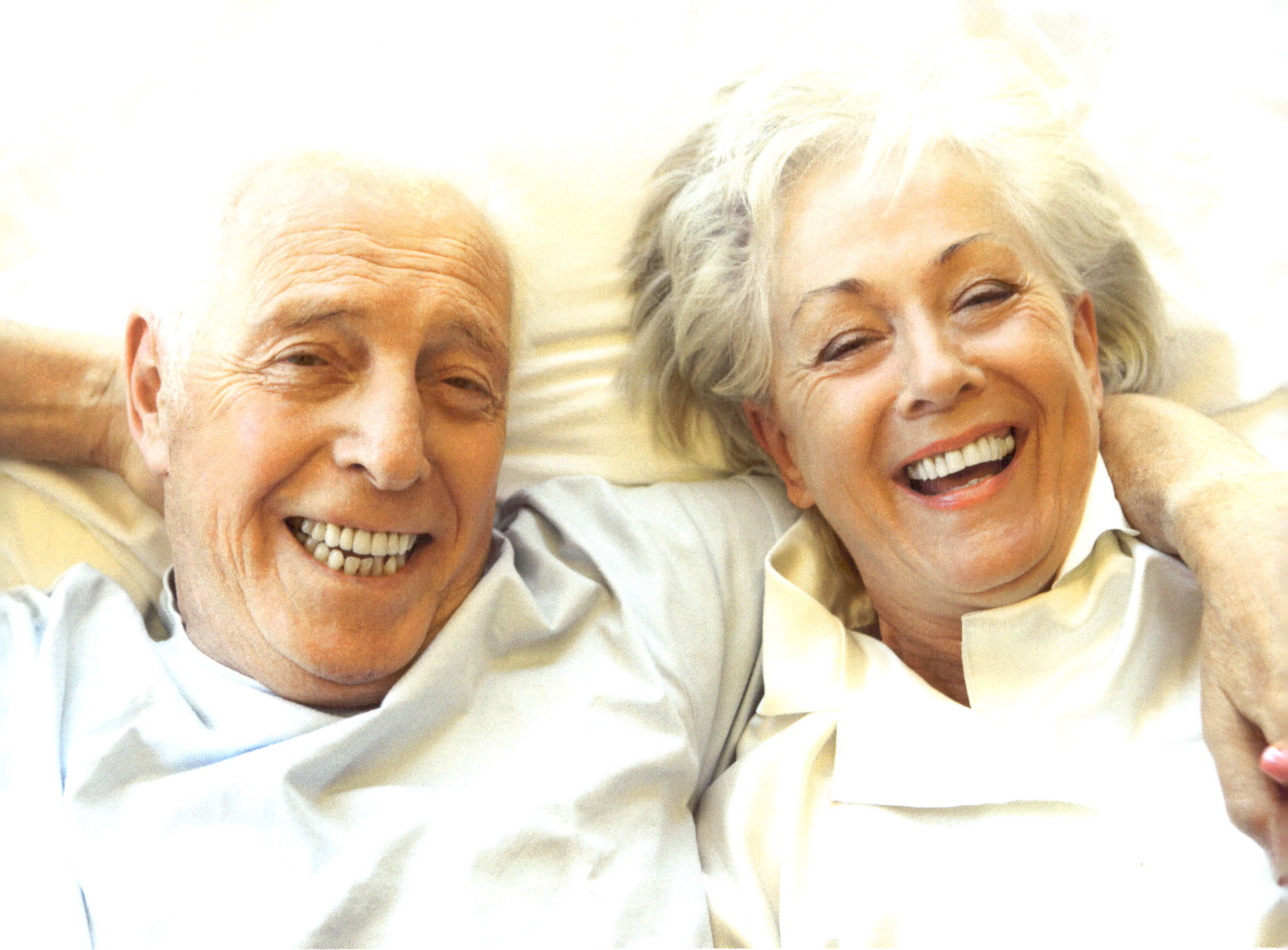

Living life fully involves communication. Perhaps one of the most perfect forms of communication is expressed by sex between two people who love each other.

It is the aim of cardiac rehabilitation and this book to remind you that life and its beauty are there for the taking. With common sense and sensible living, you can again do most, if not all, of the things you enjoy. This includes the most special function of the heart, the act of loving.

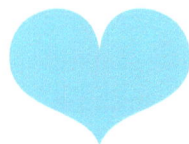

Notes

---

www.ingramcontent.com/pod-product-compliance
Lightning Source LLC
Chambersburg PA
CBHW060855270326
41934CB00002B/154